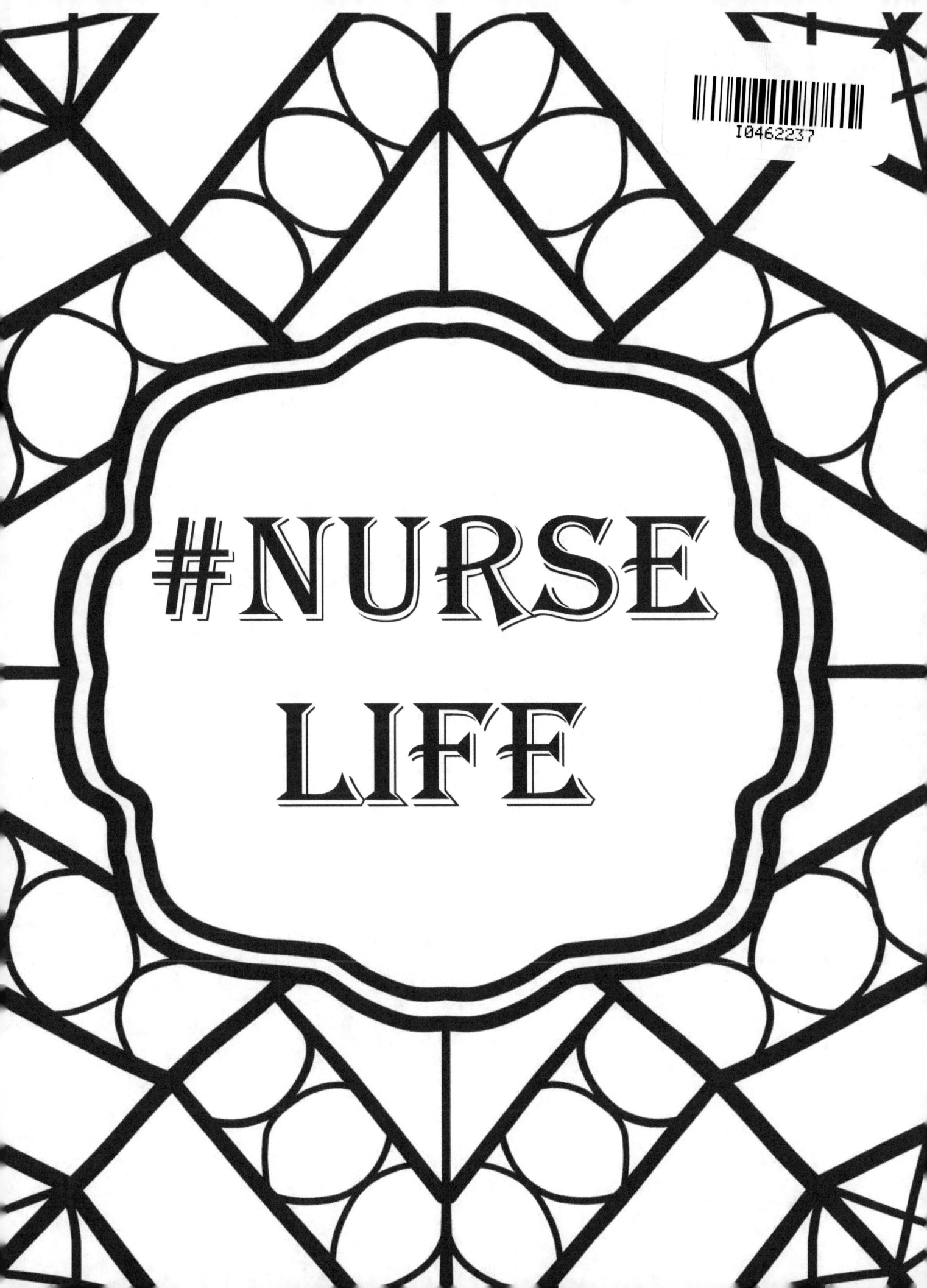

#NURSE LIFE

Ativan A Nurse's Best Friend

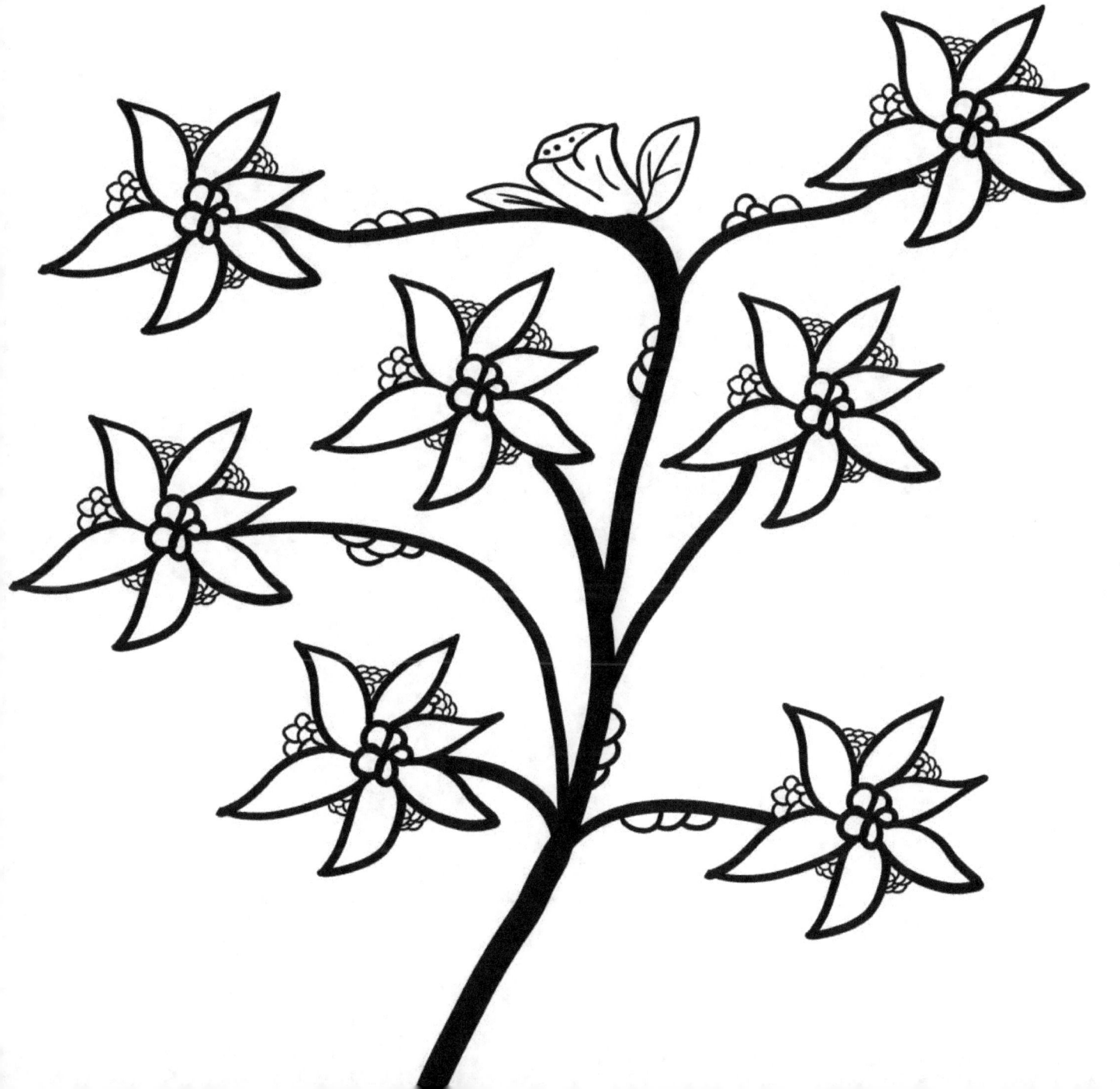

Best Nurse Ever

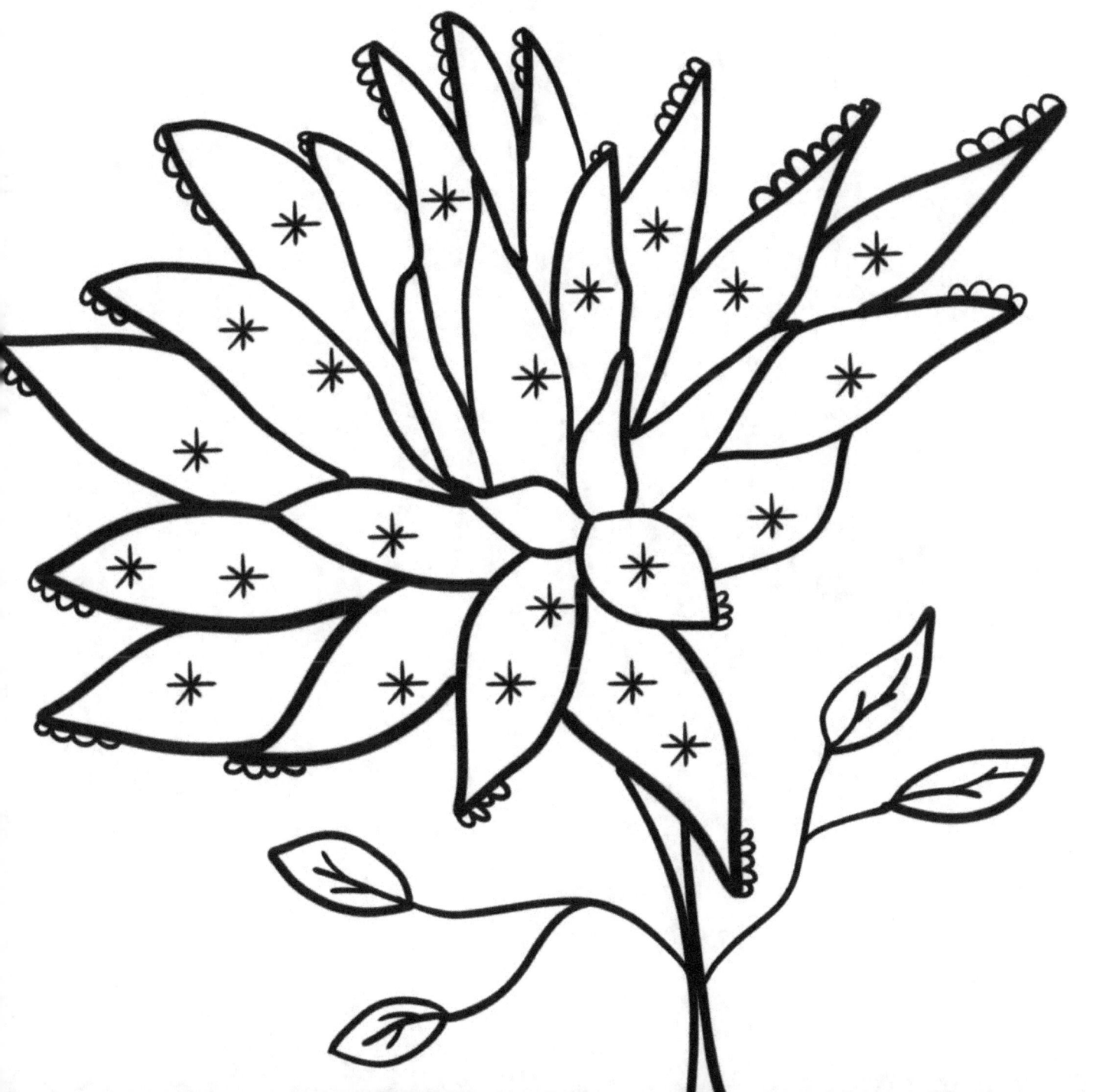

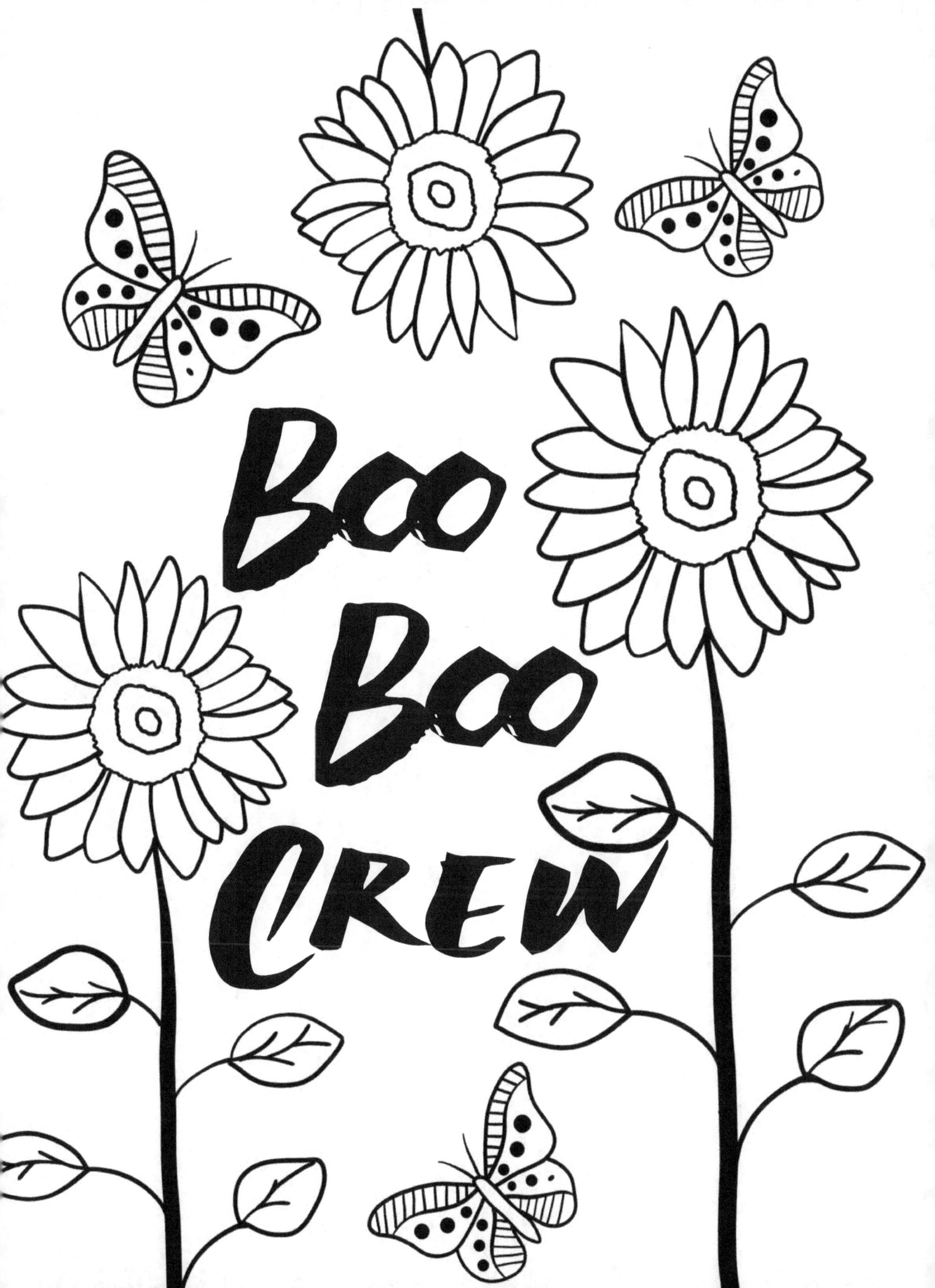

Coffee Scrubs Rubber Gloves

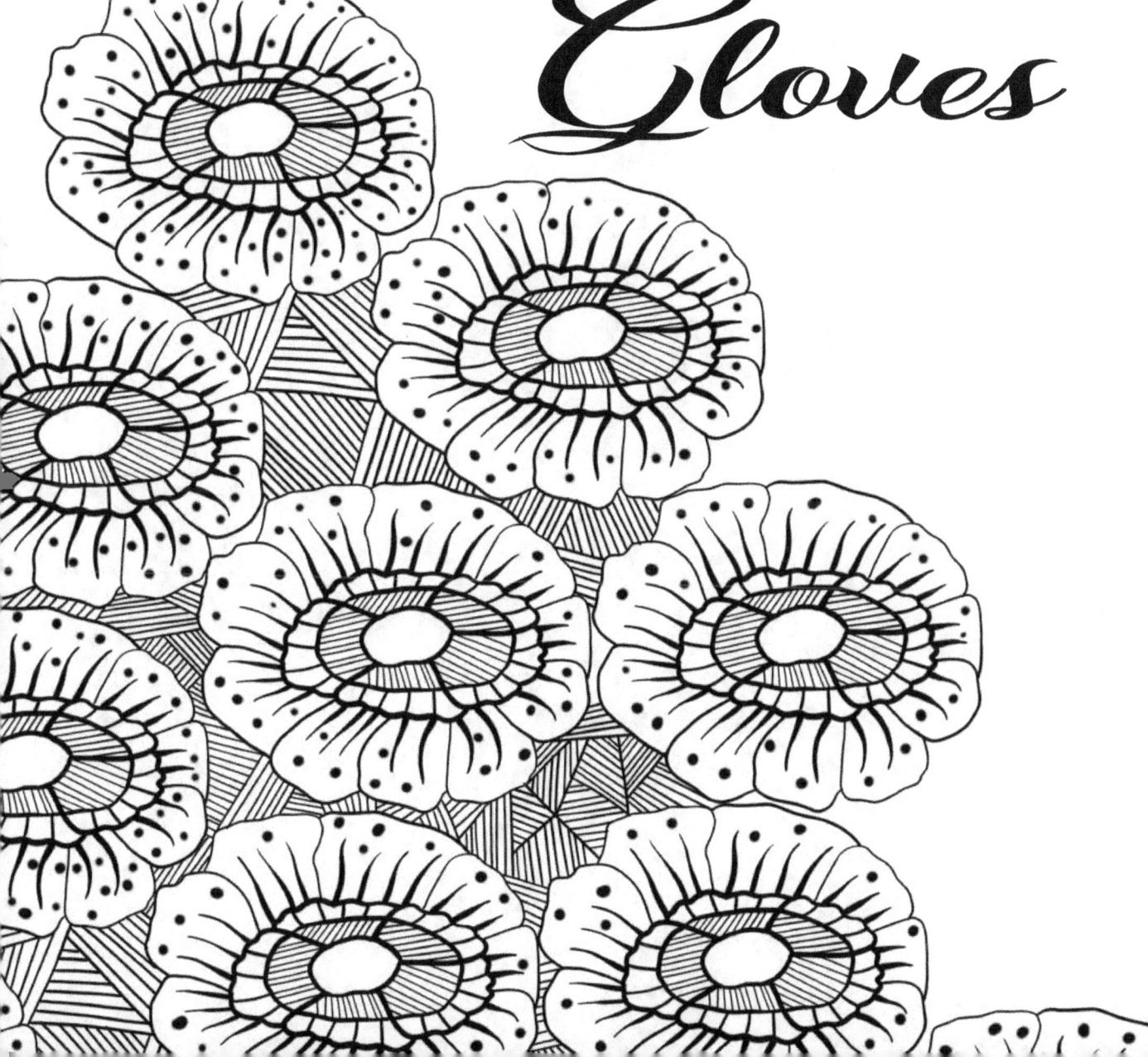

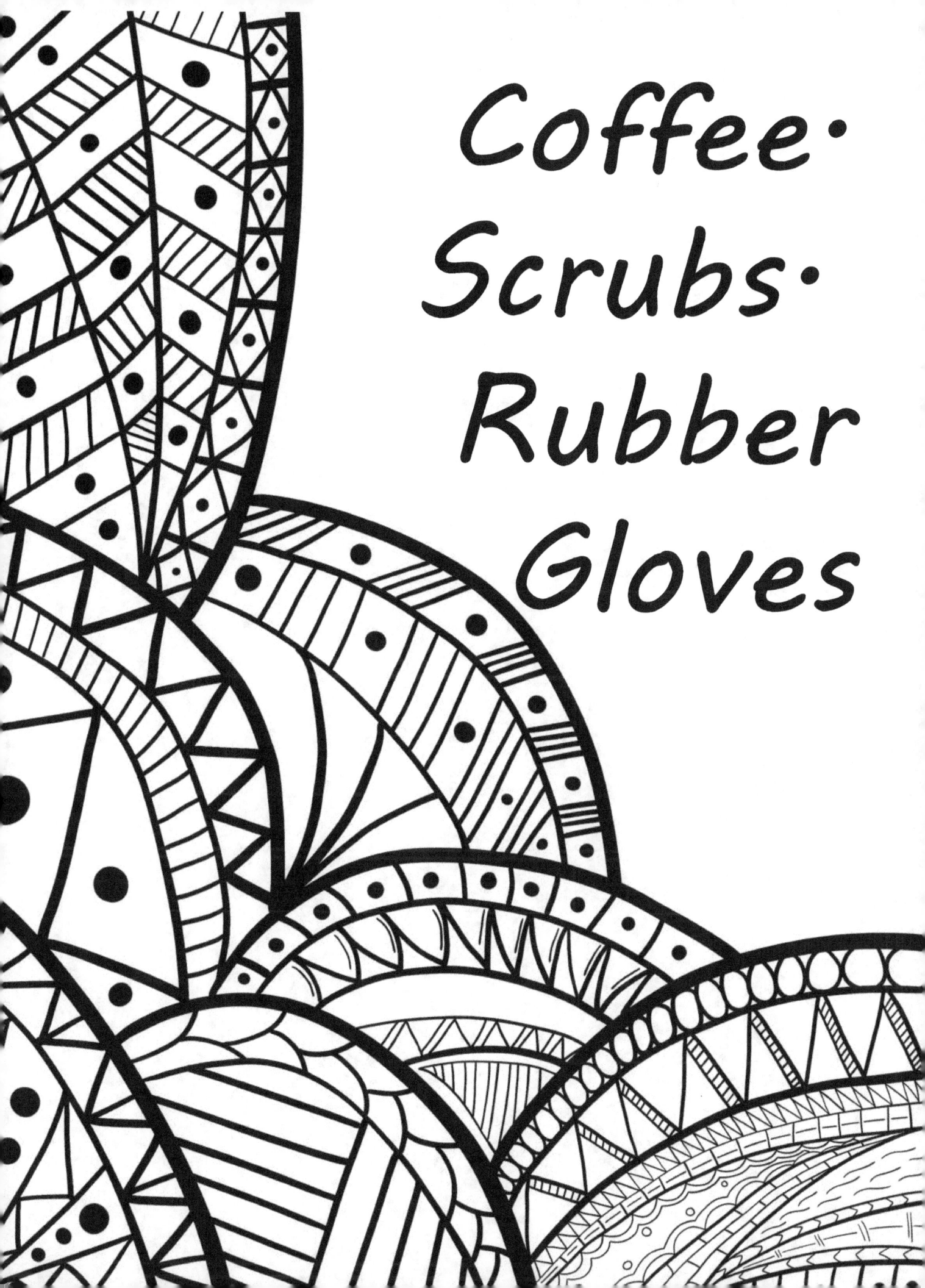

Coffee·
Scrubs·
Rubber
Gloves

DO NOT MAKE ME SEDATE YOU.

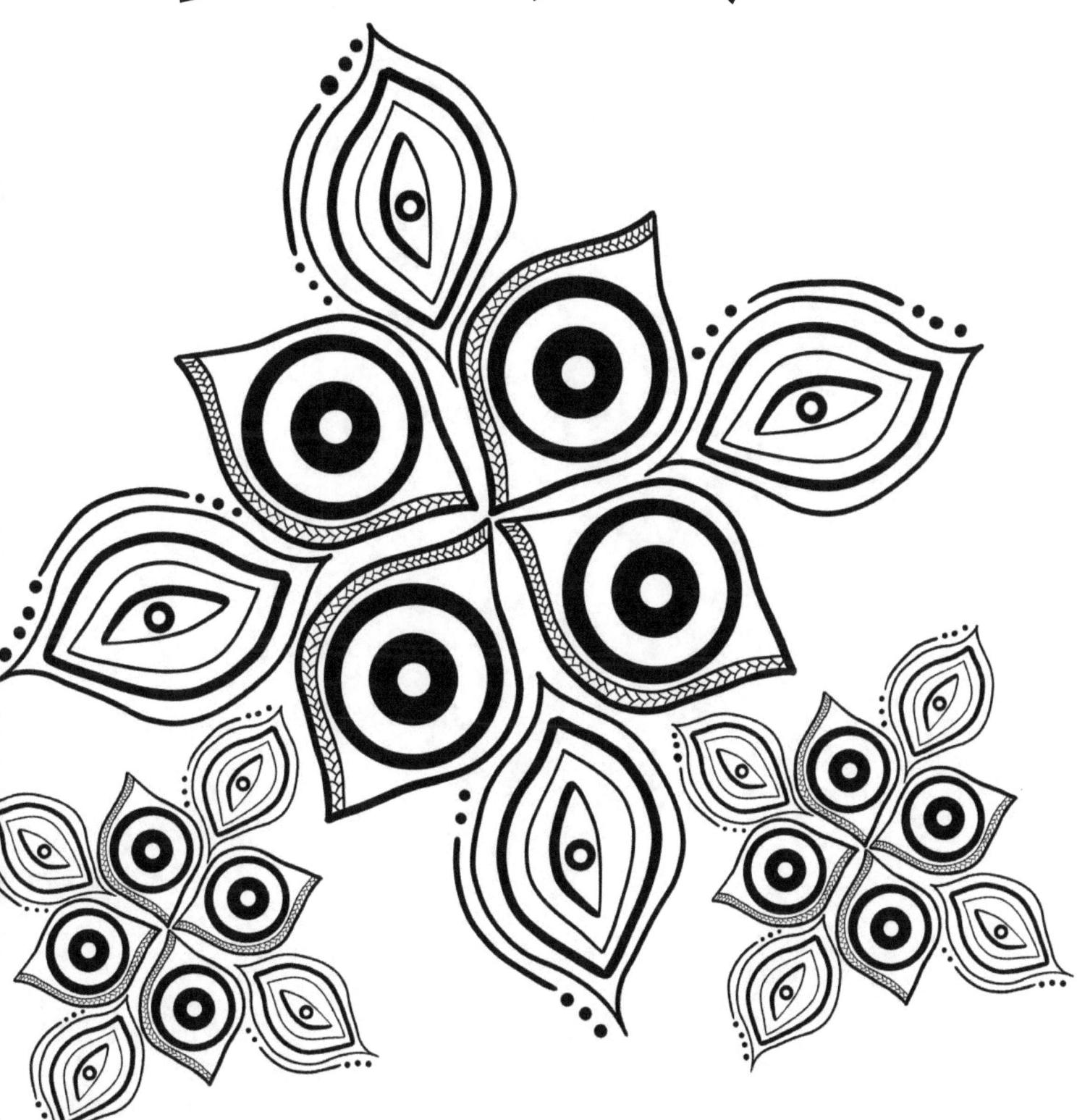

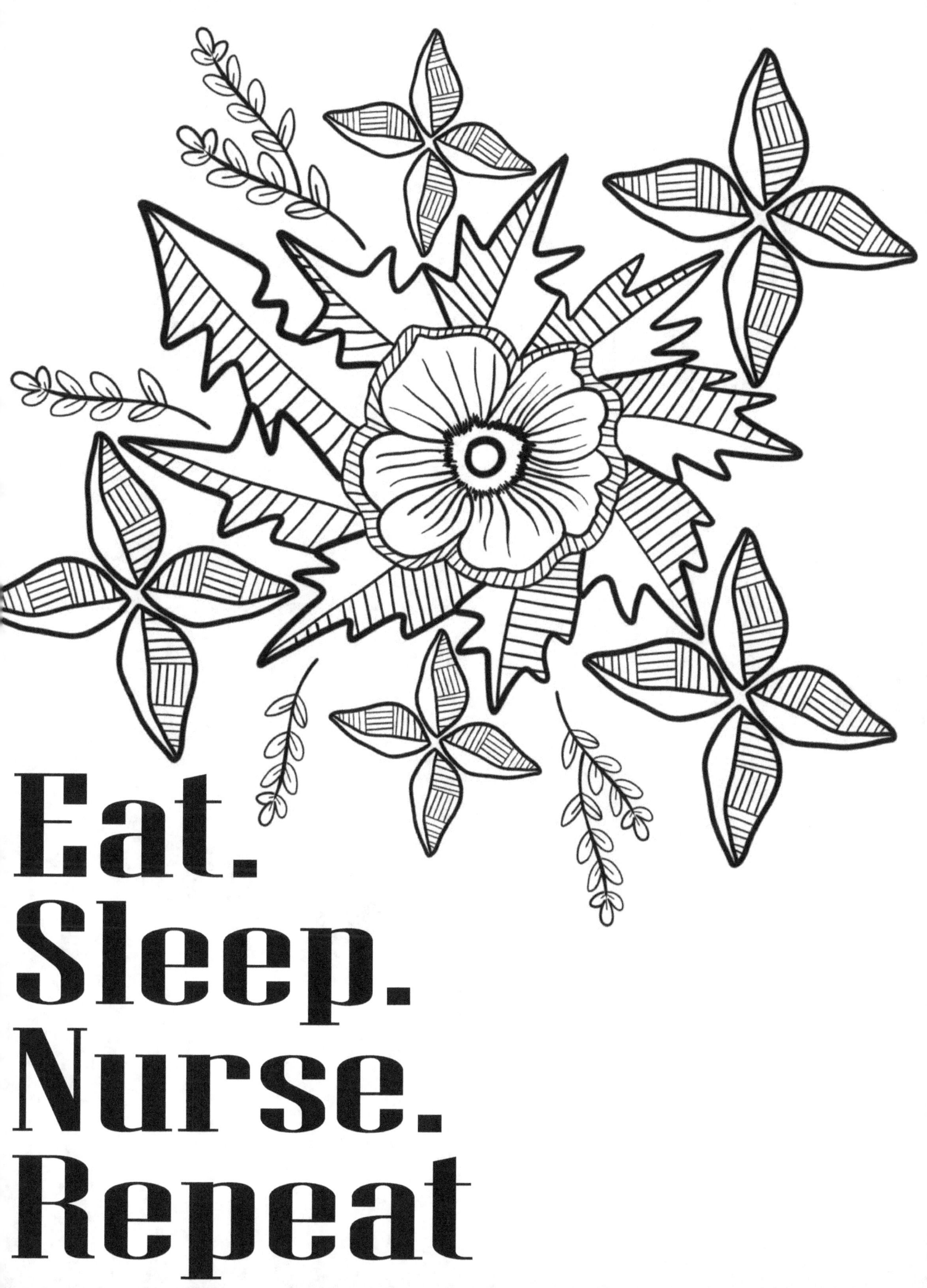

Eat.
Sleep.
Nurse.
Repeat

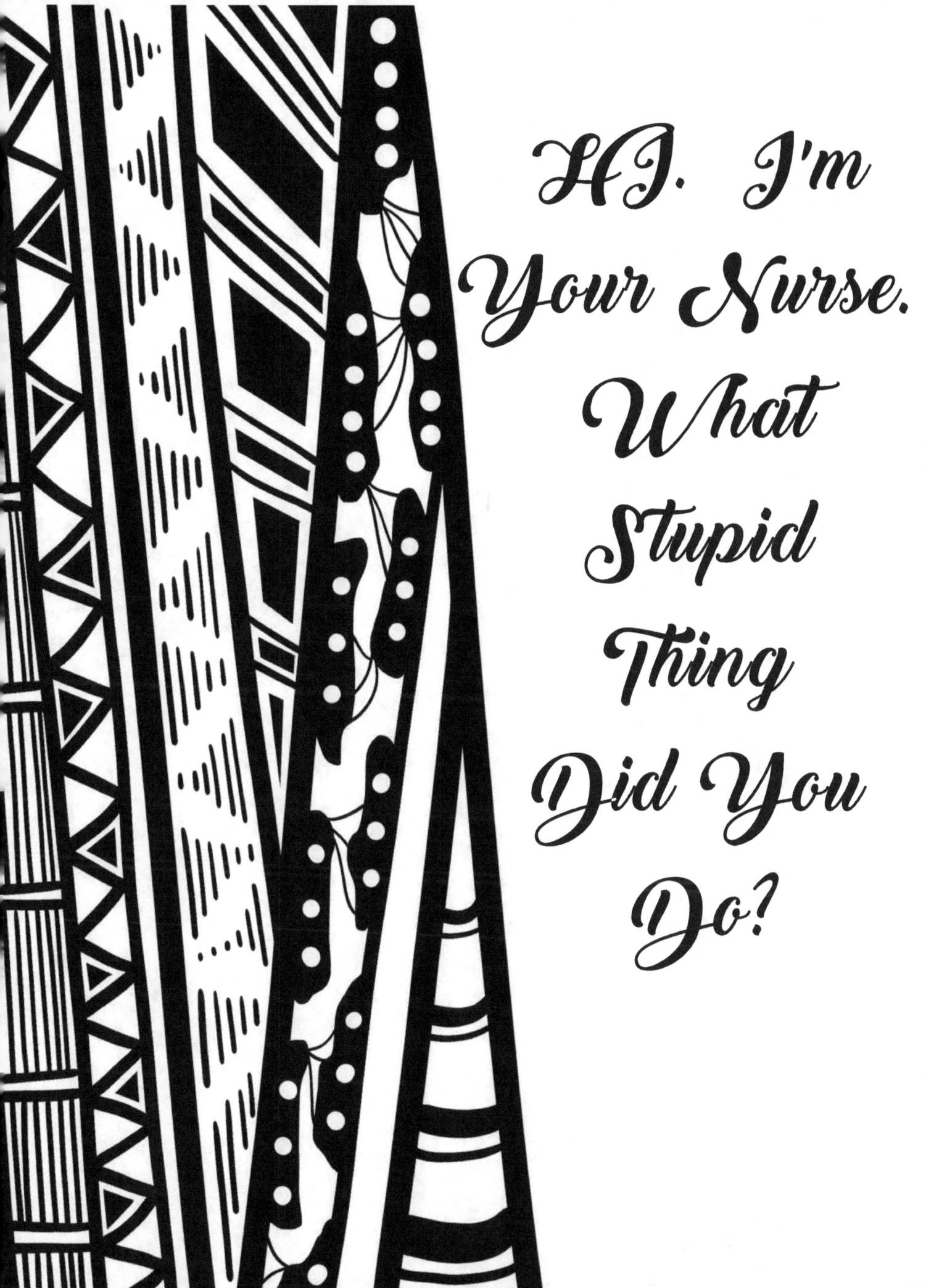

I Call The Shots

WISH THERE WAS A CURE FOR STUPID

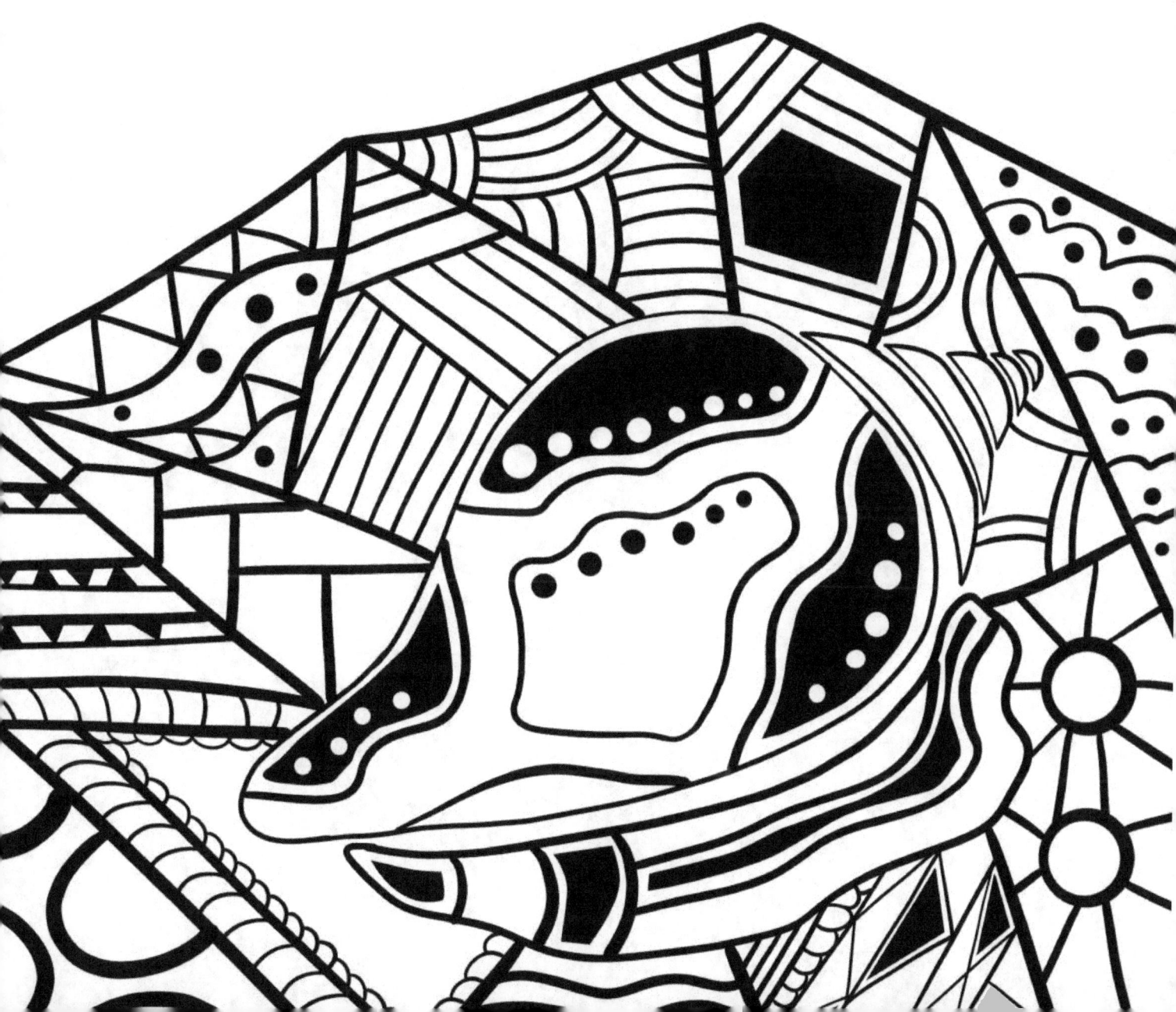

I'm Just Here For The Card Game

I'VE SEEN IT, SMELLED IT, TOUCHED IT, HEARD IT, AND STEPPED IN IT

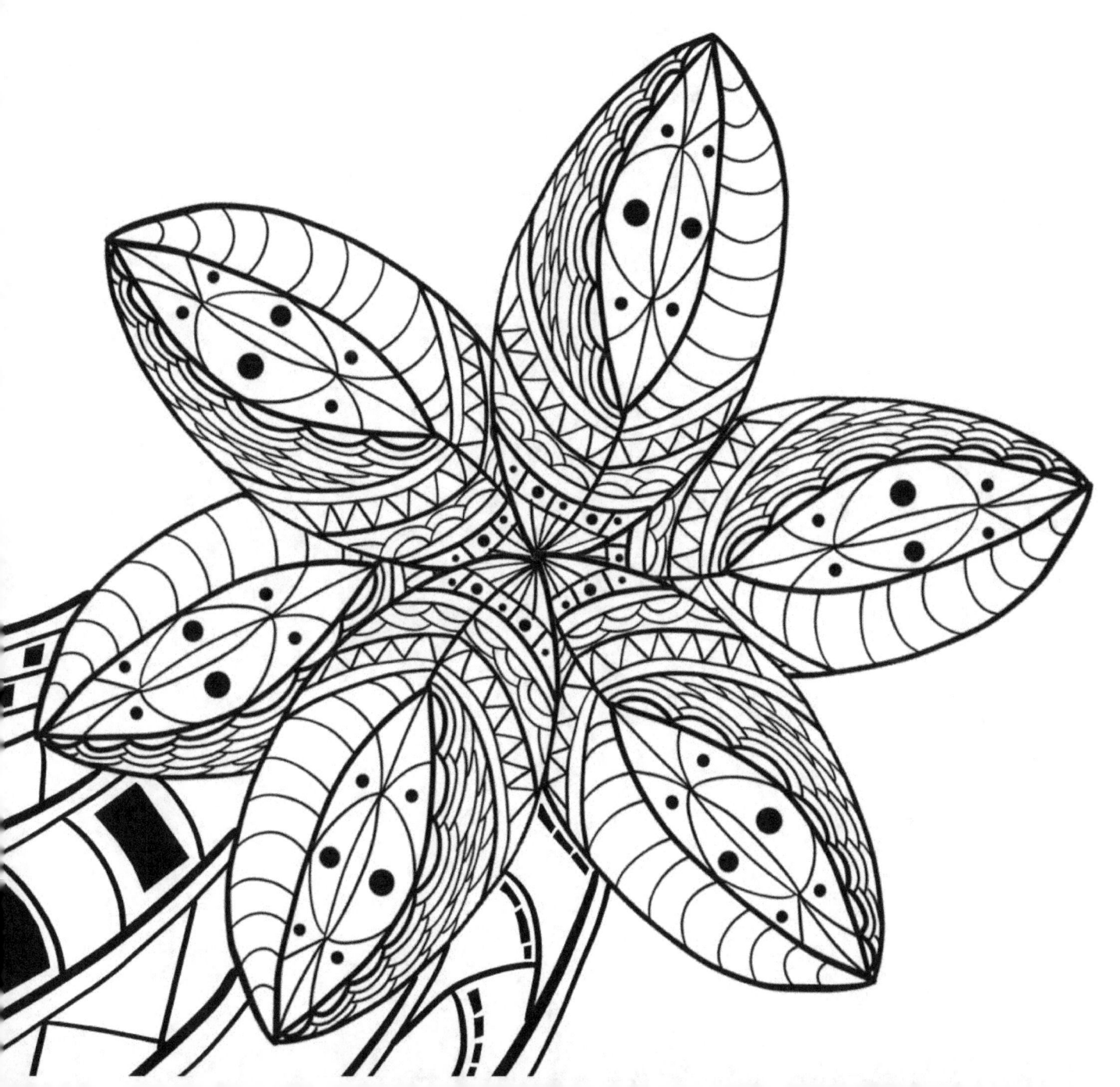

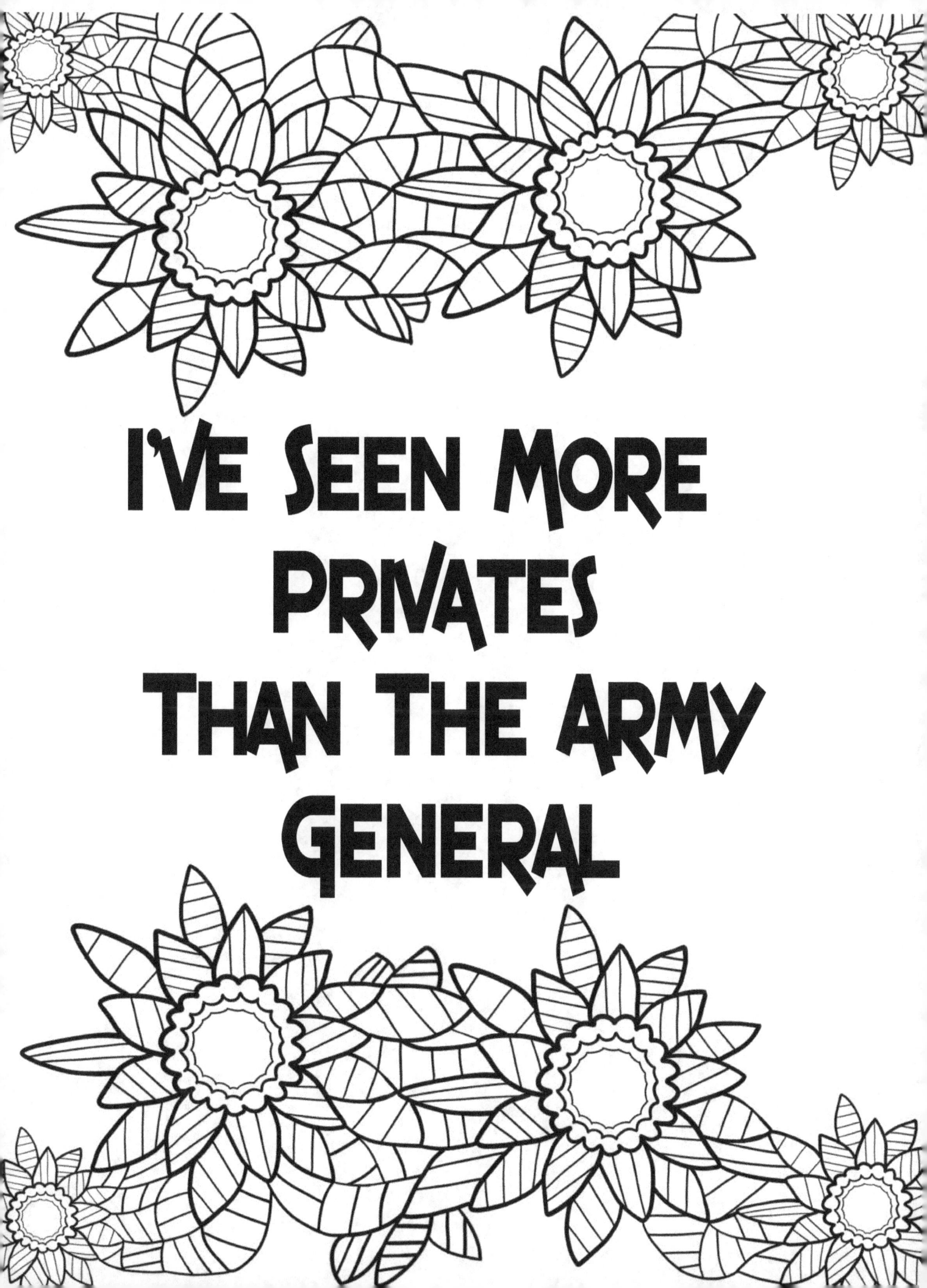

I'VE SEEN MORE PRIVATES THAN THE ARMY GENERAL

If You're Happy and You Know It, It's Your Meds

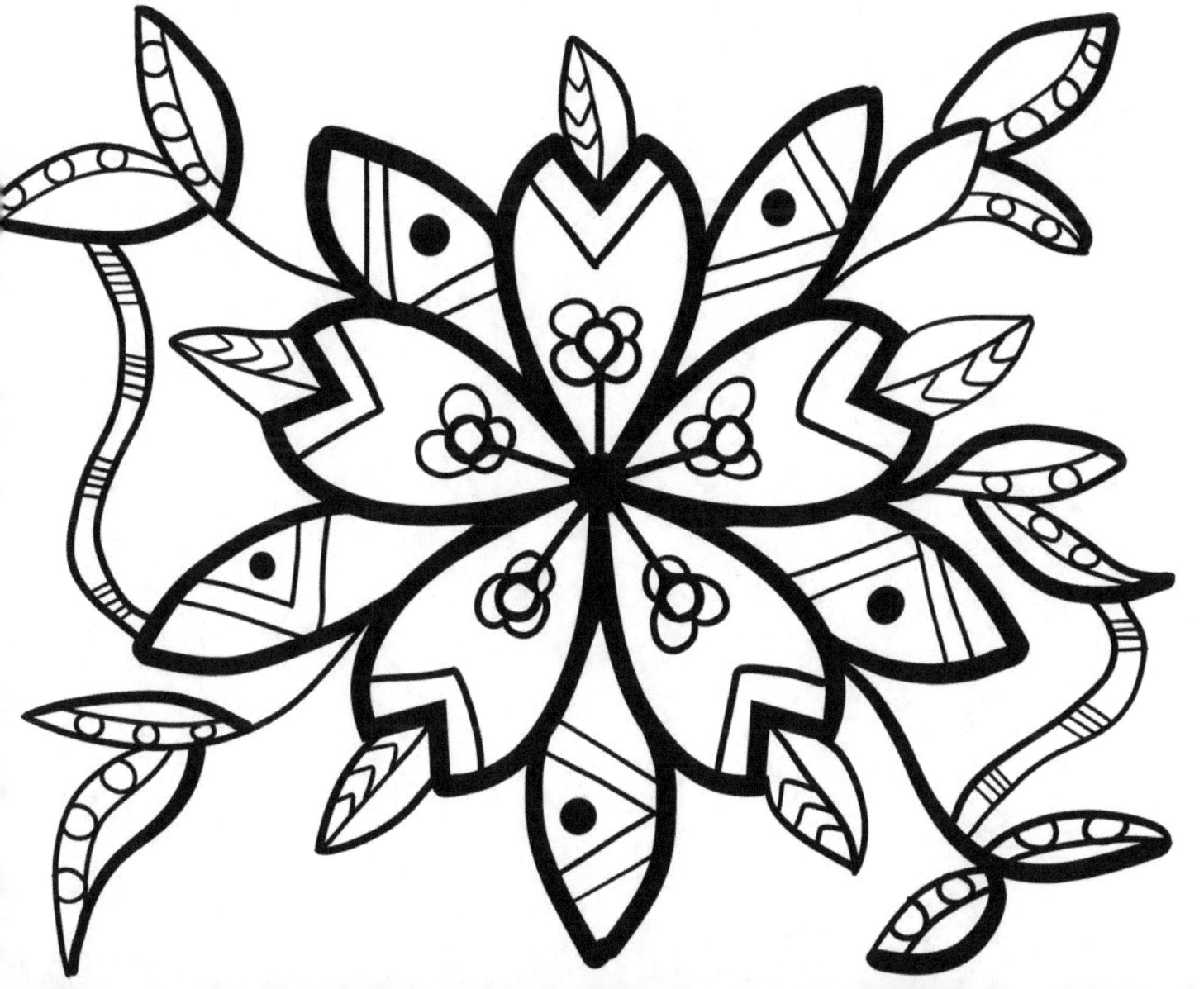

IT'S A NURSE THING. YOU WOULDN'T UNDERSTAND

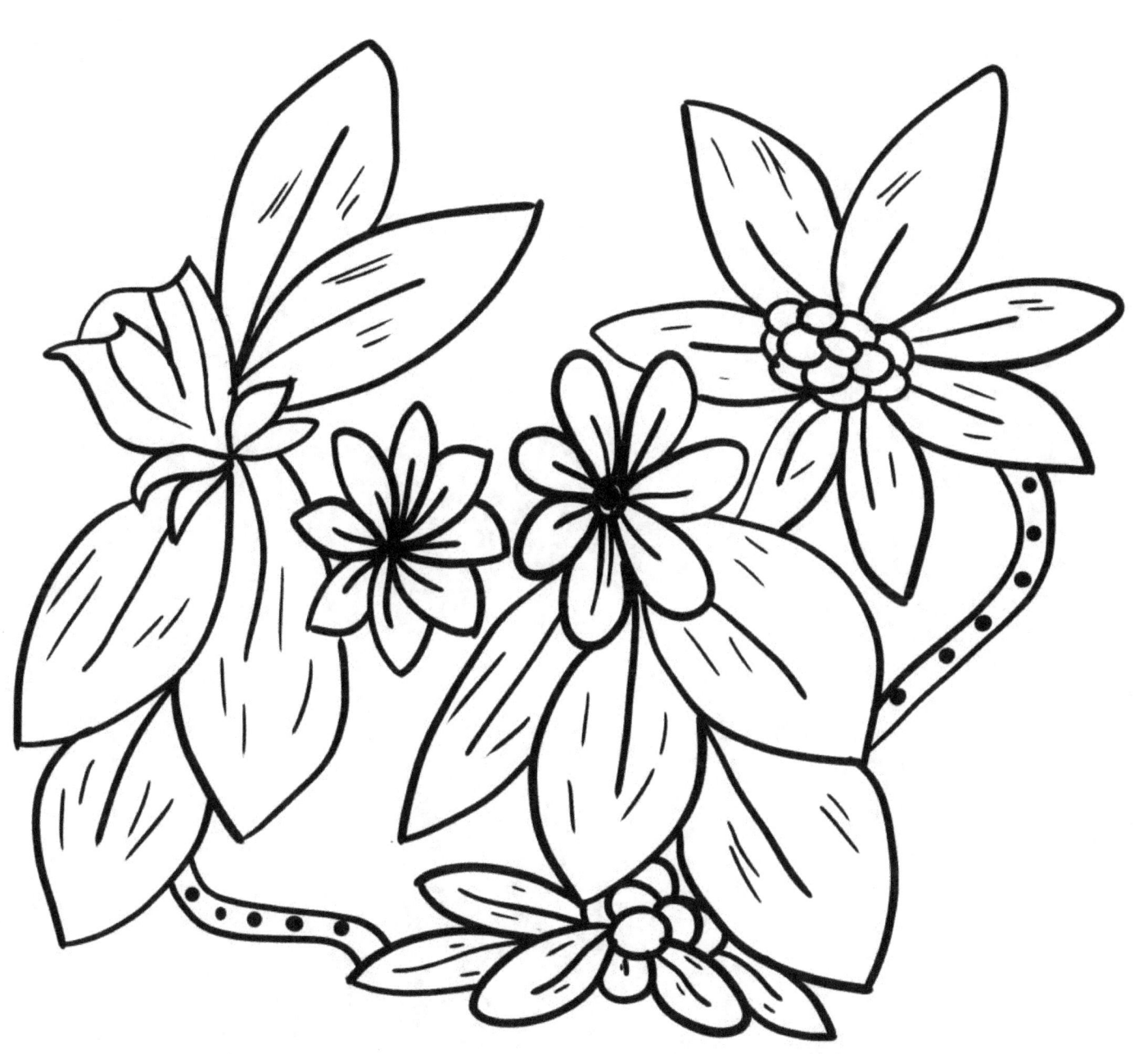

Multitasking, Life-Saving, Miracle Worker

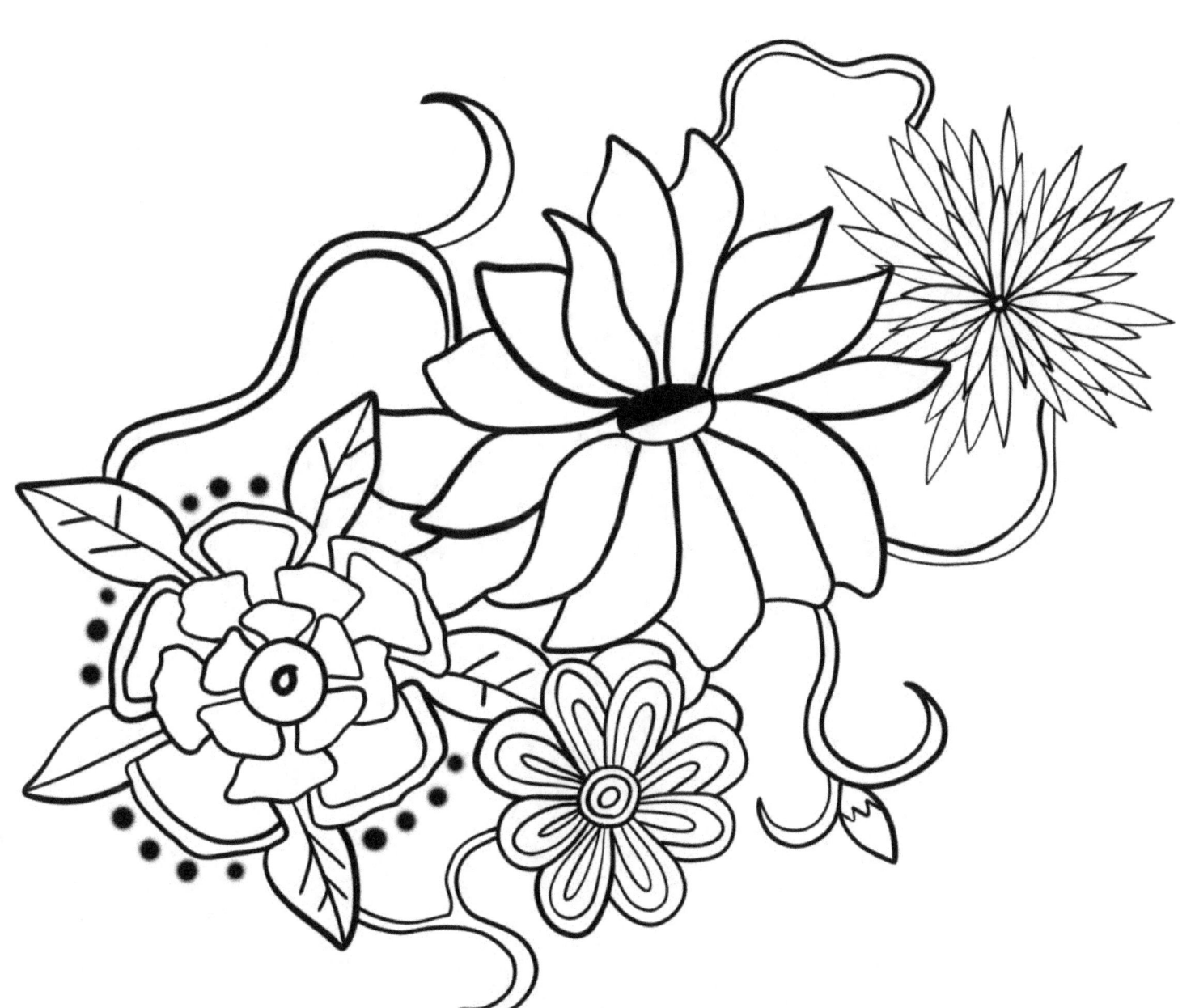

N.U.R.S.E. I'LL BE THERE FOR YOU

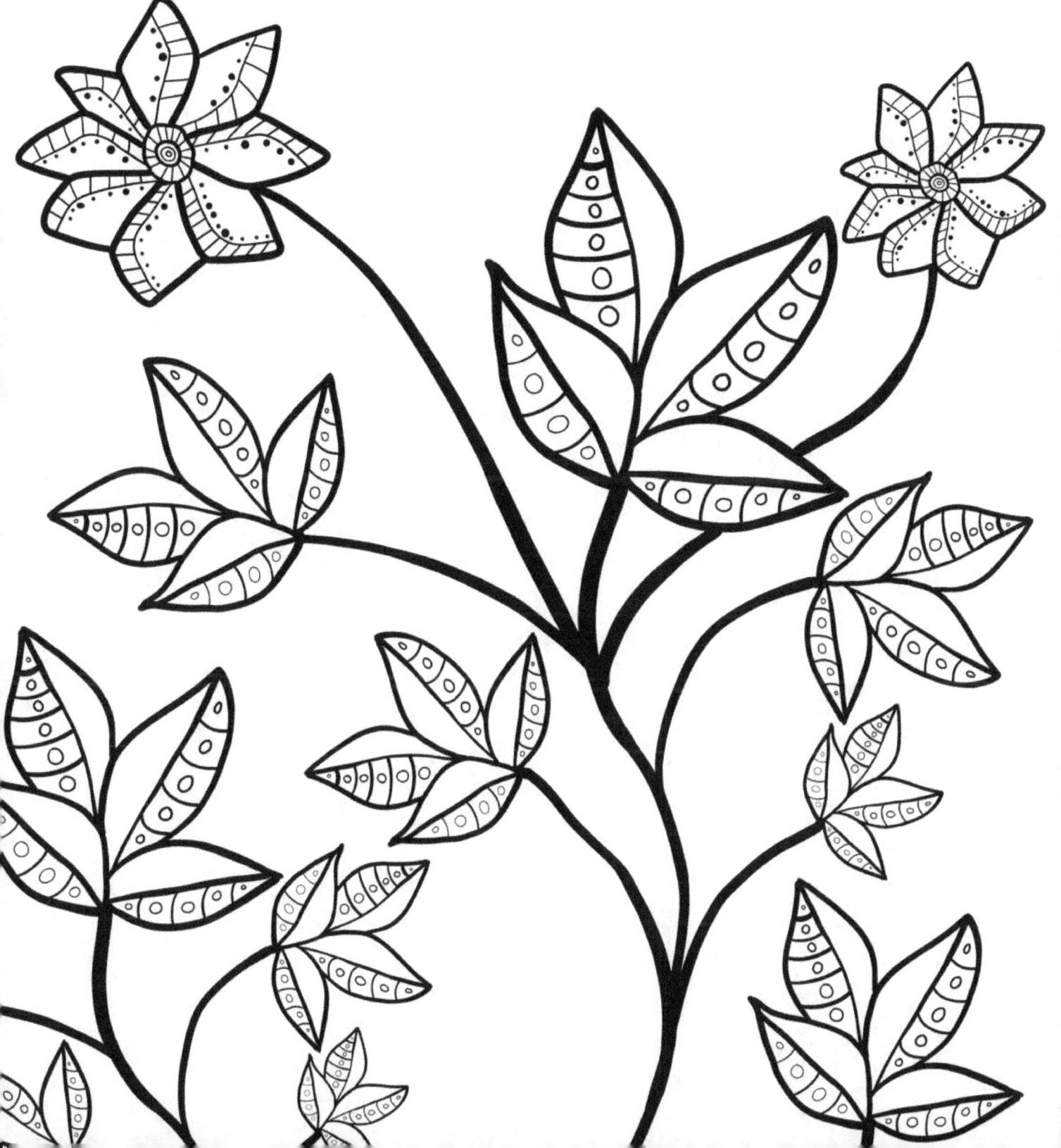

Nurse Squad

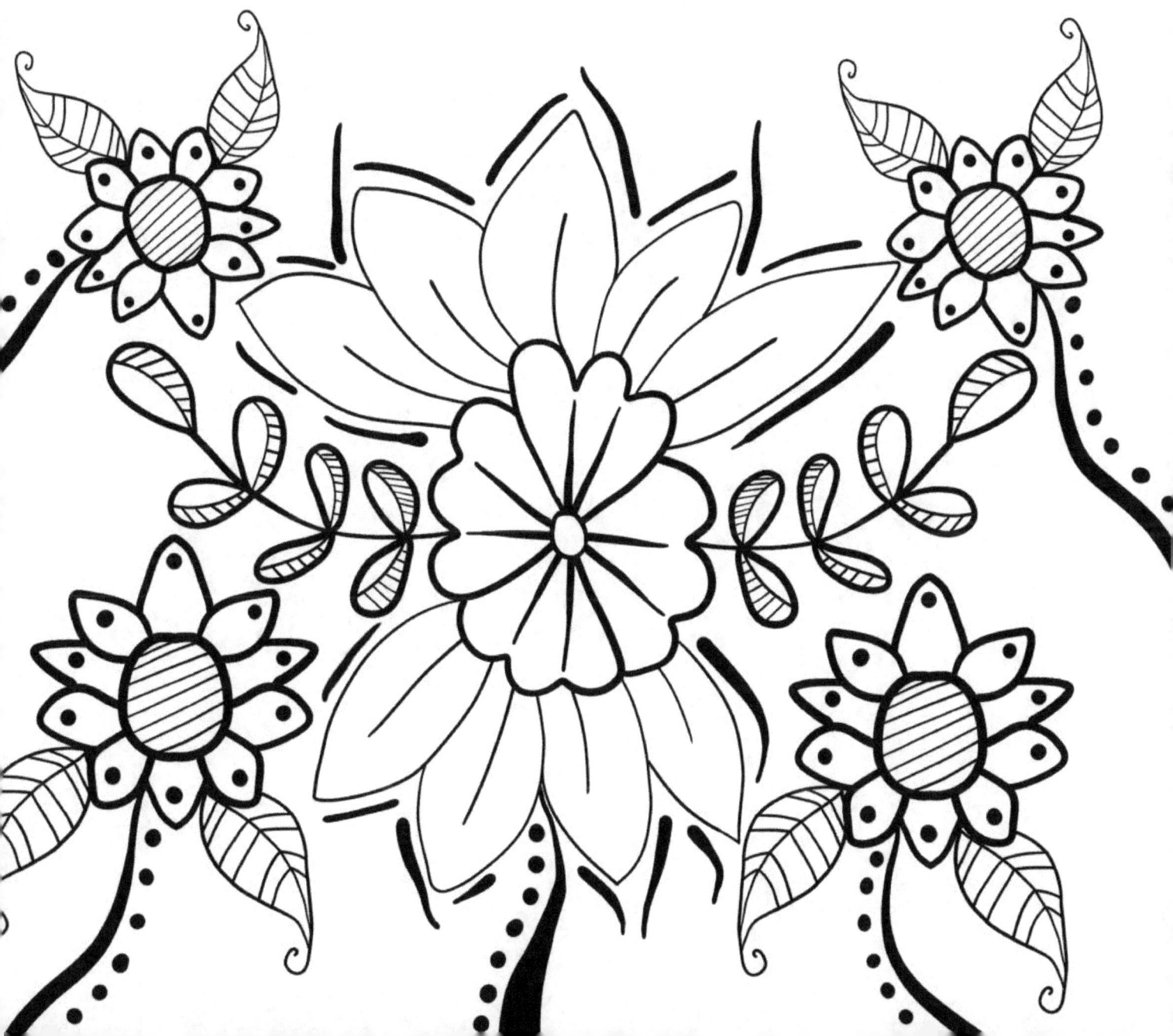

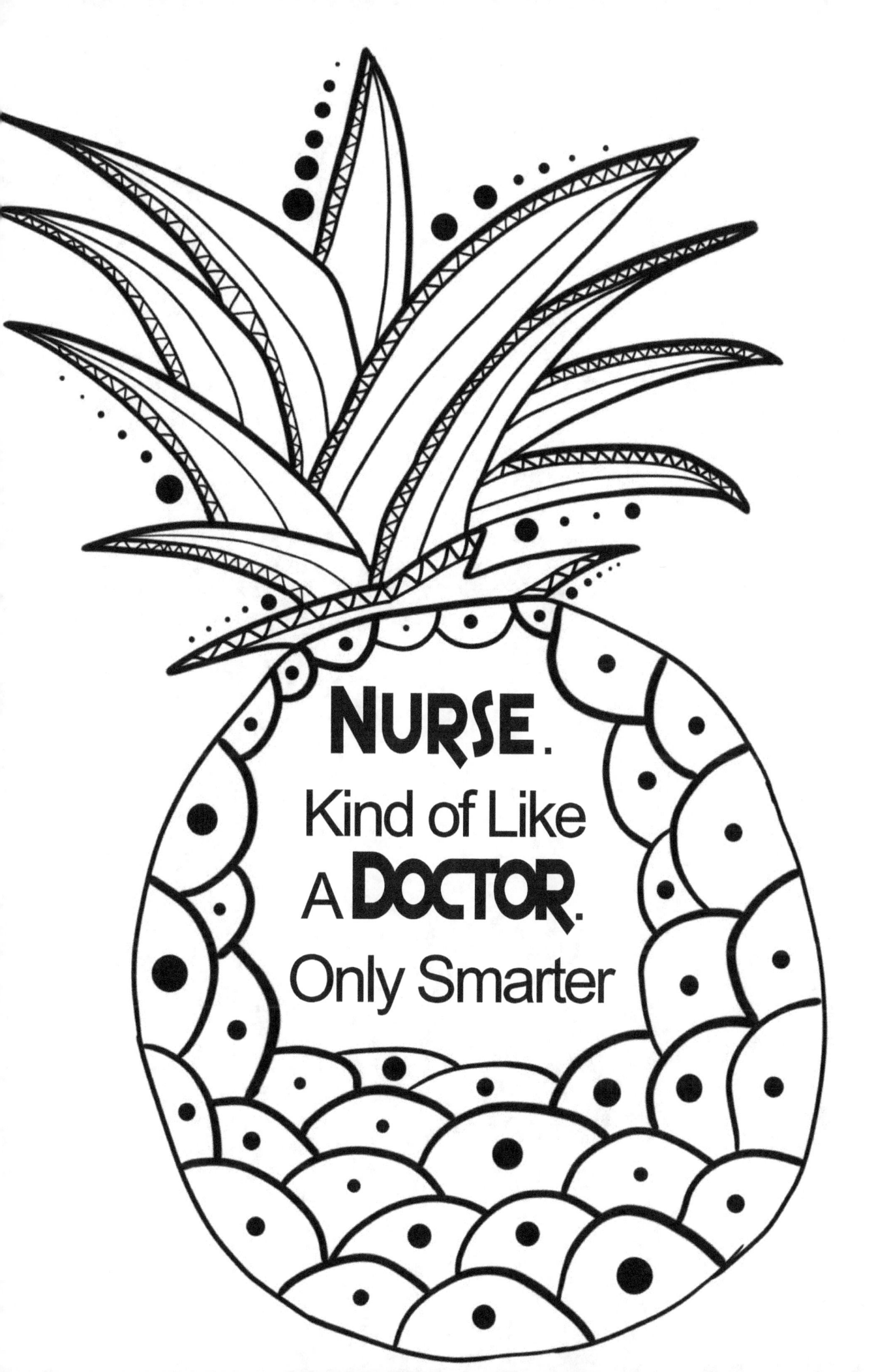

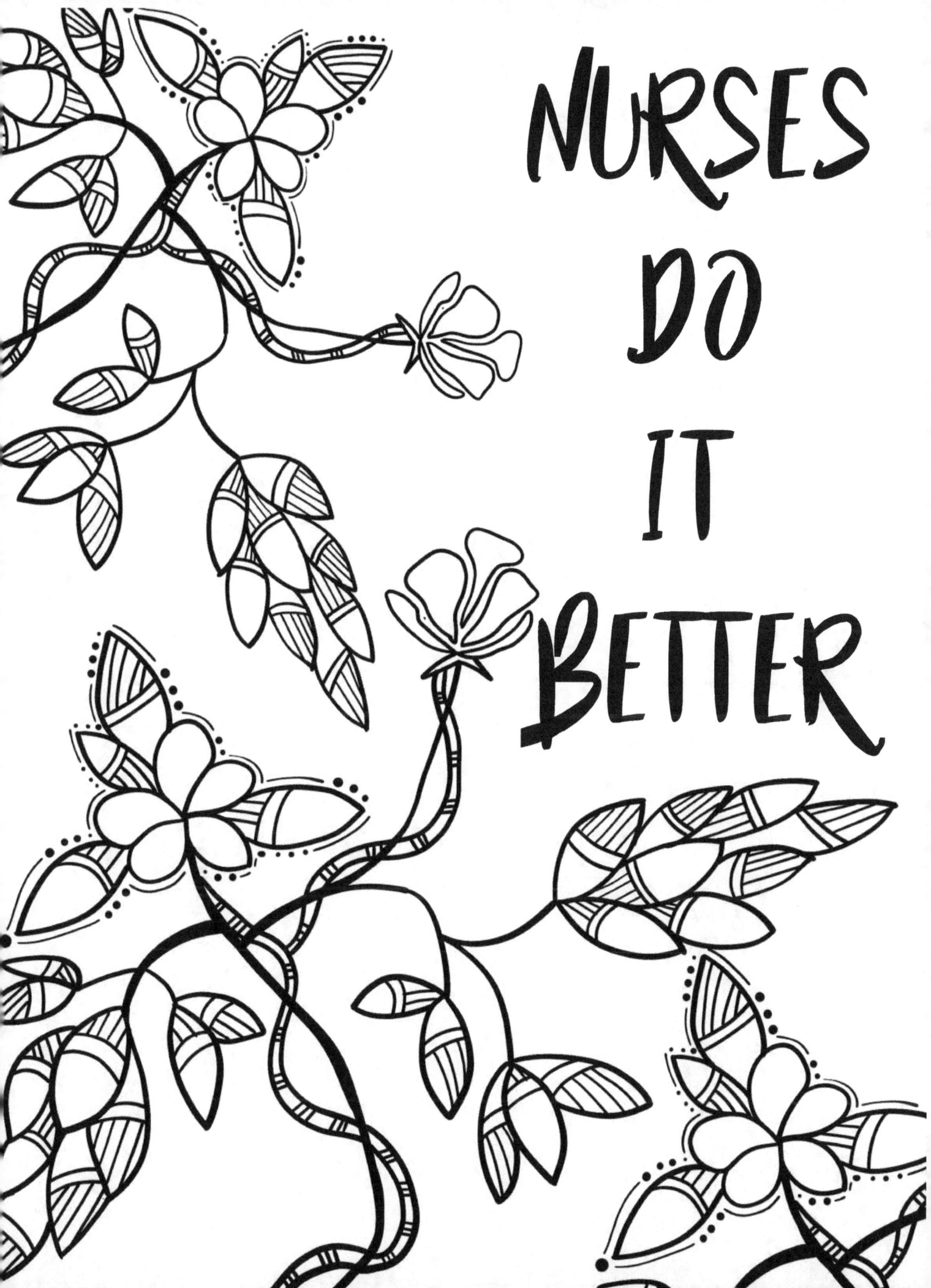

NURSES DO IT BETTER

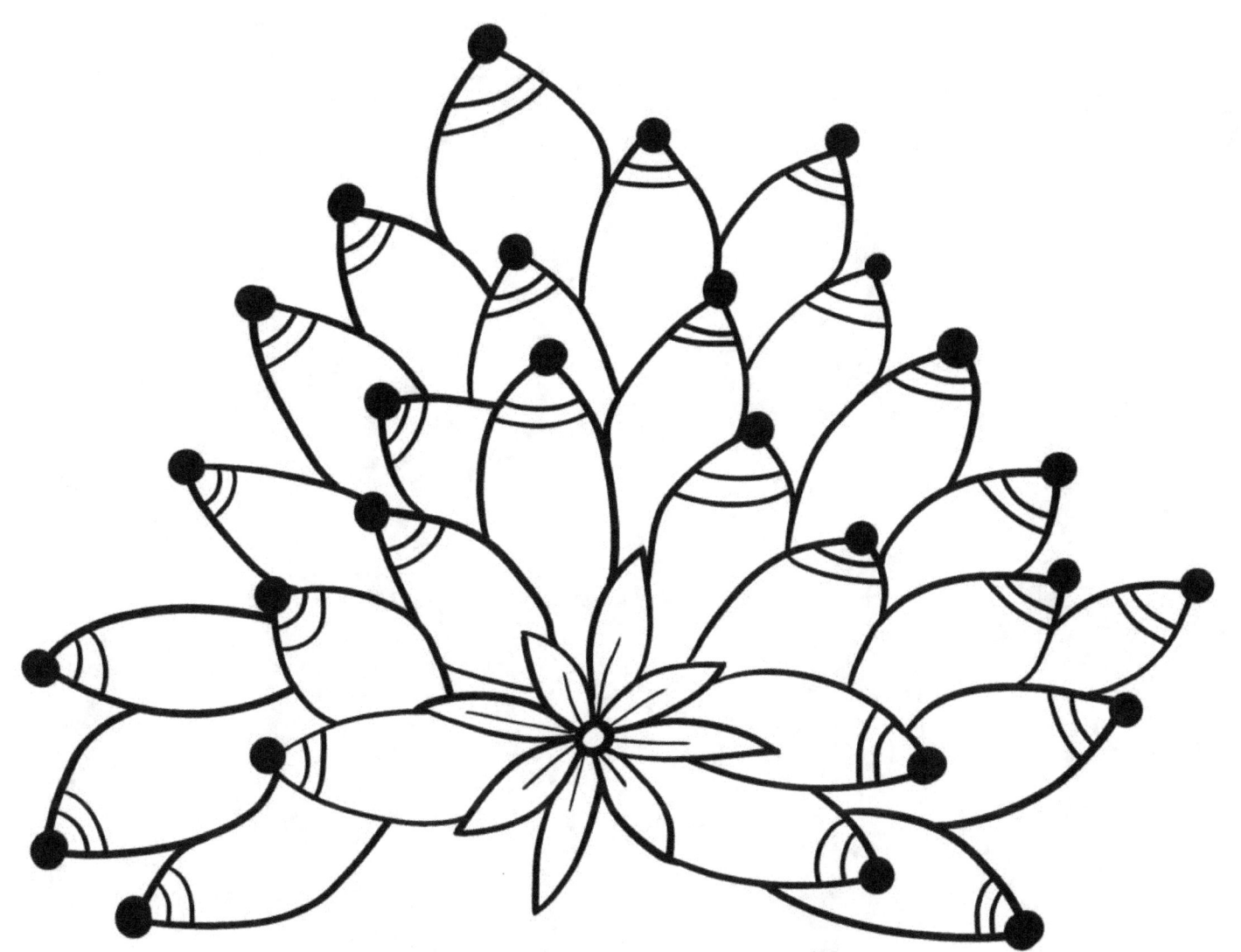

NURSING 10%
PATIENT CARE,
90%
DOCUMENTATION

PRN Does Not Mean Please Remind The Nurse

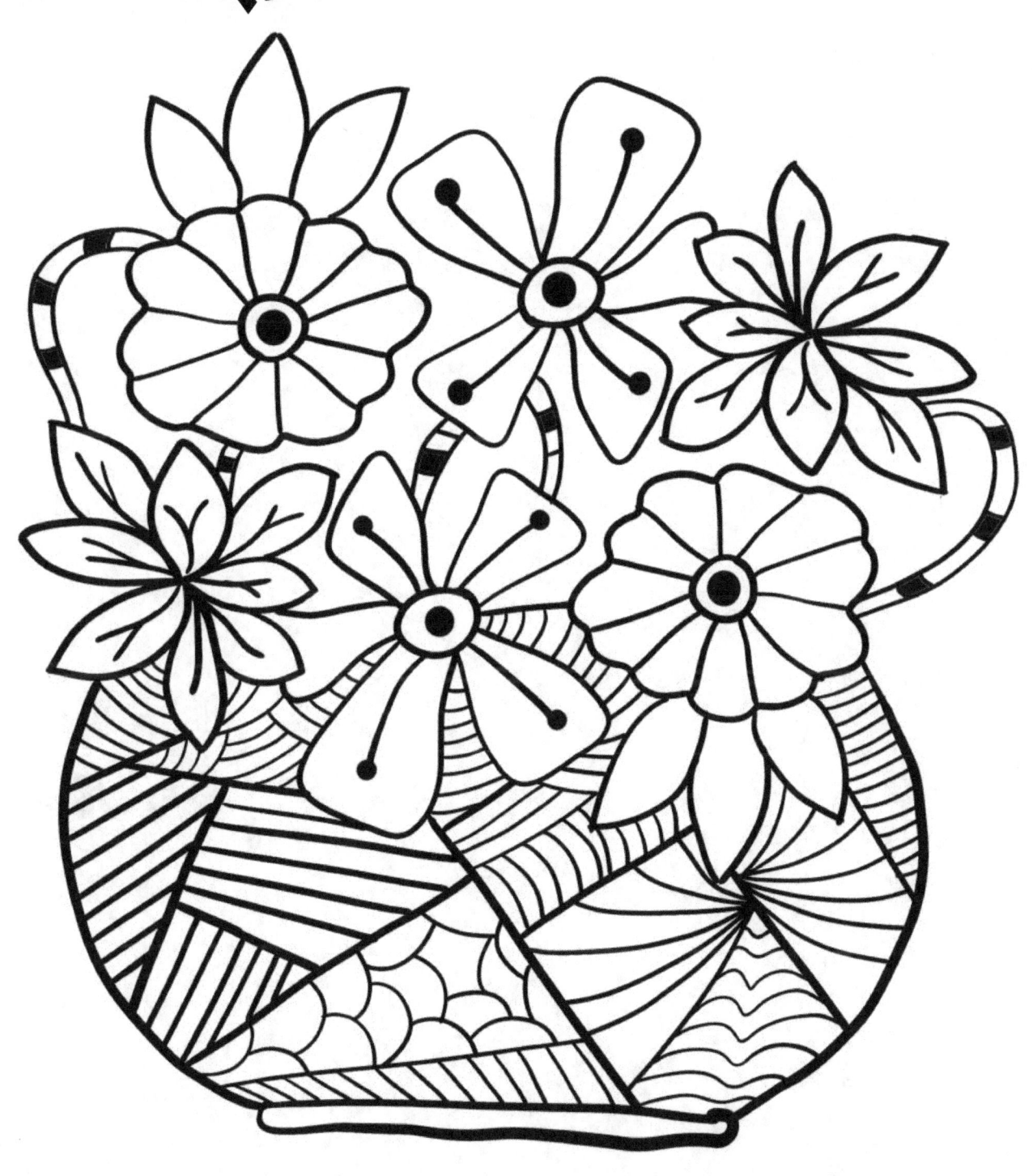

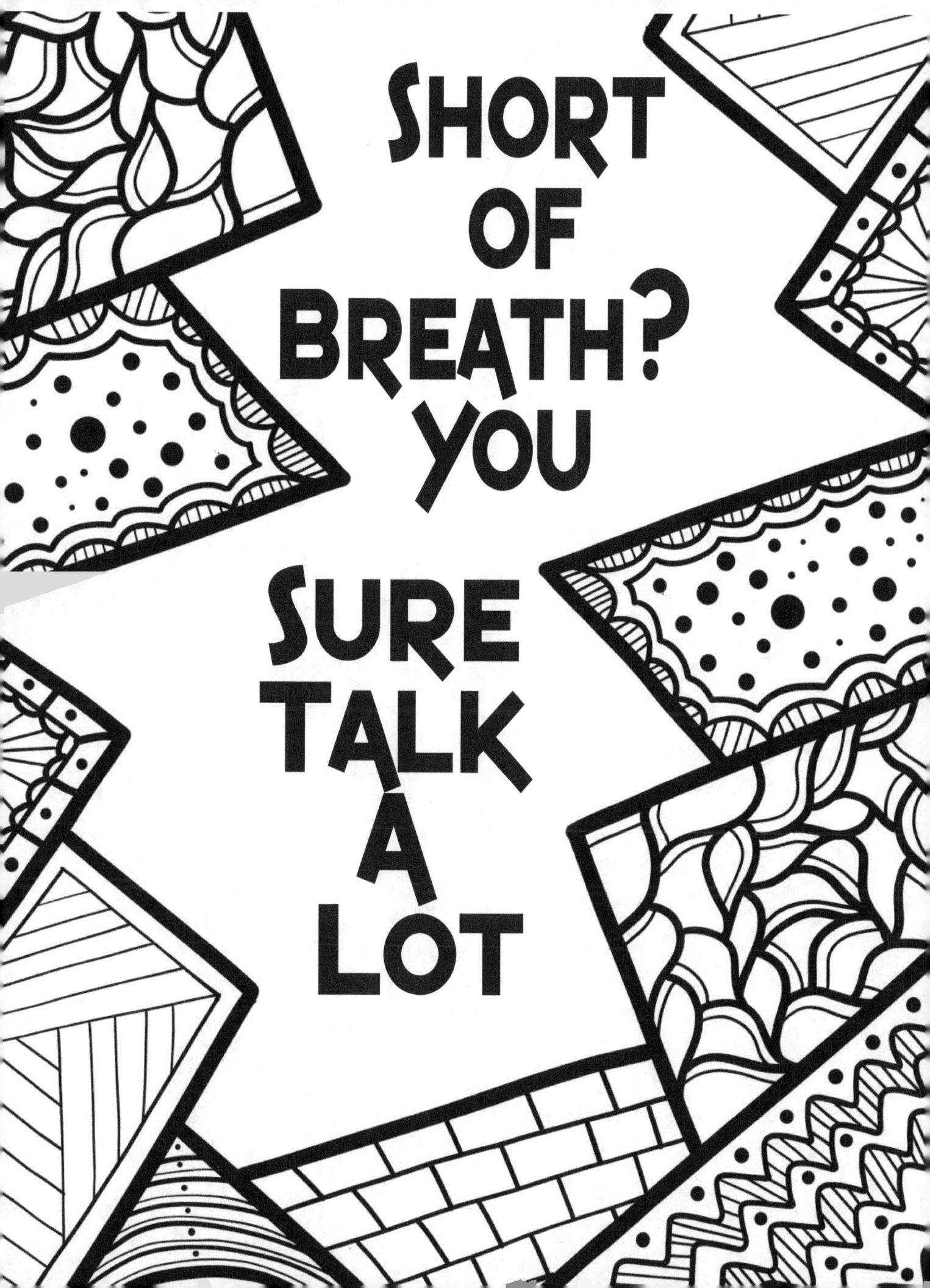

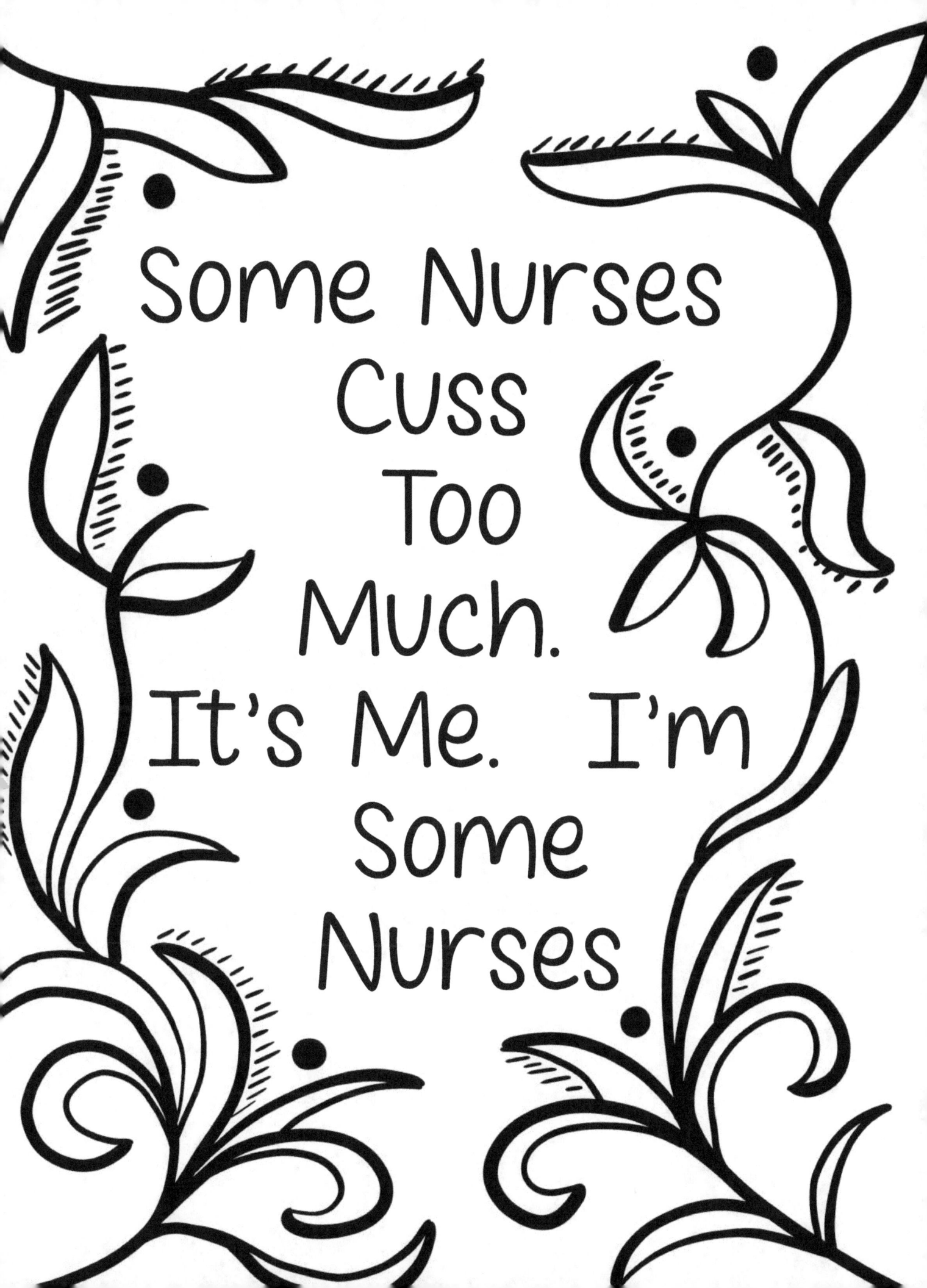

Some Nurses Cuss Too Much. It's Me. I'm Some Nurses

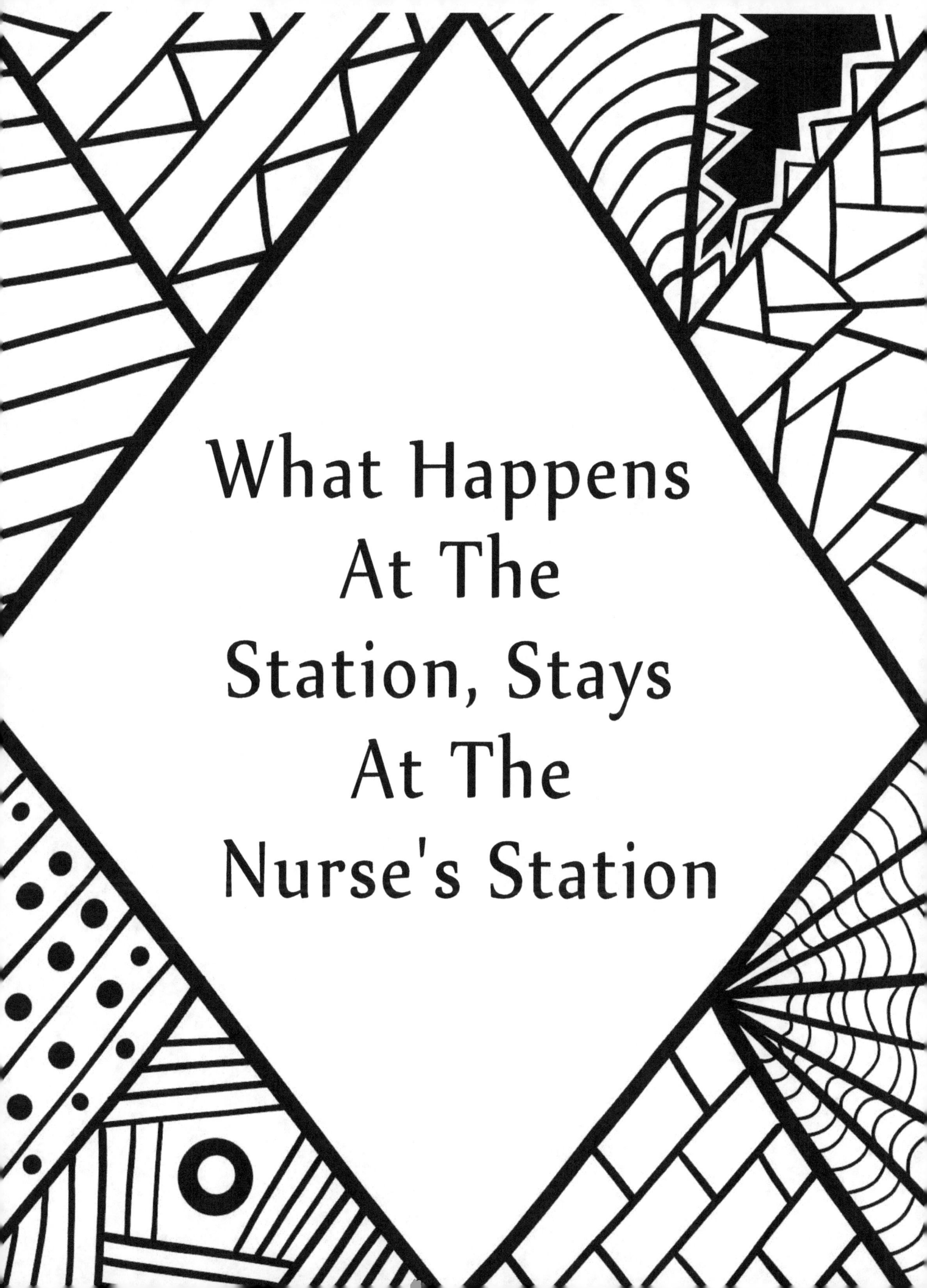

What Happens
At The
Station, Stays
At The
Nurse's Station

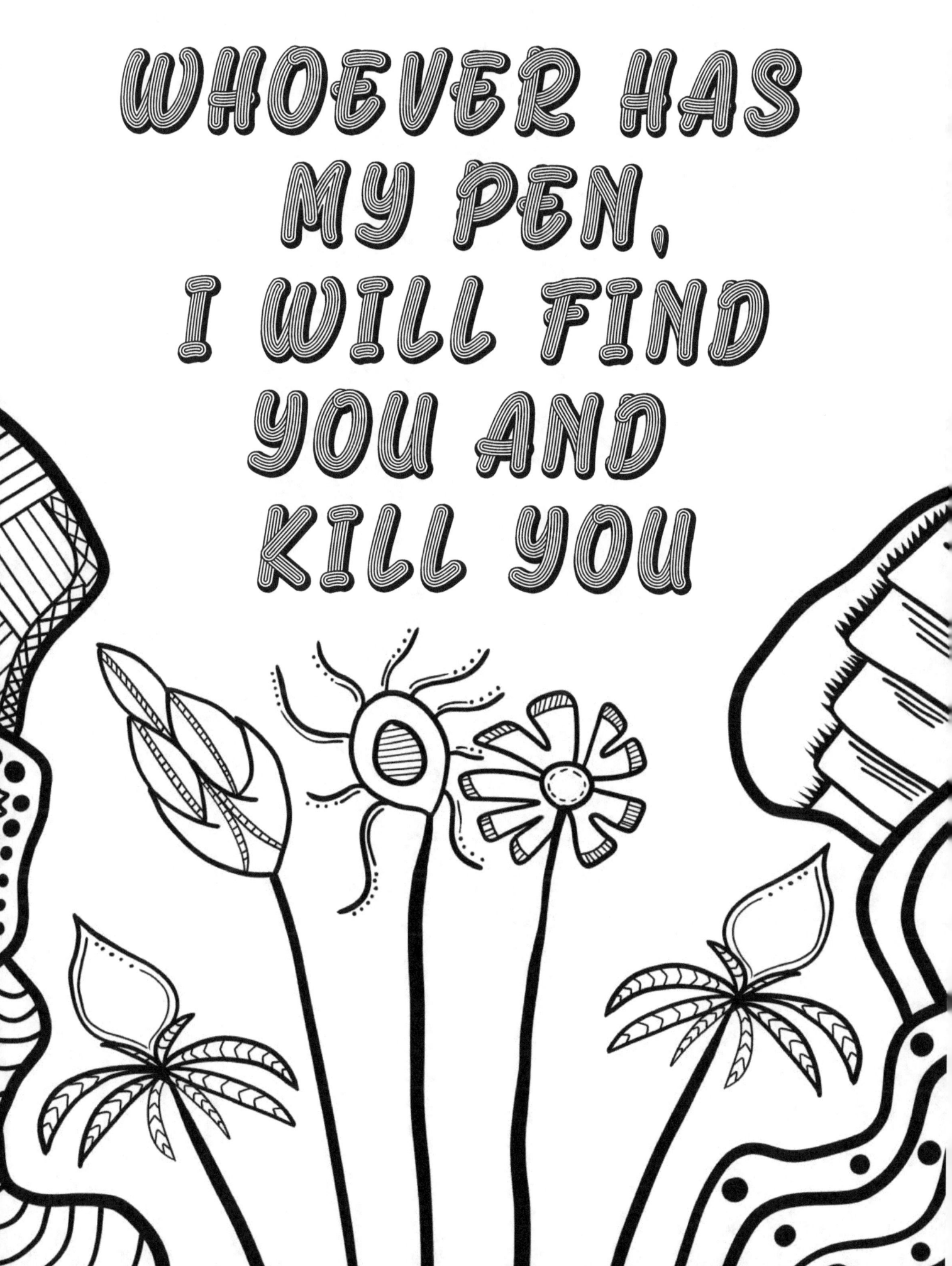

WILL GIVE MEDICAL ADVICE FOR CHOCOLATE

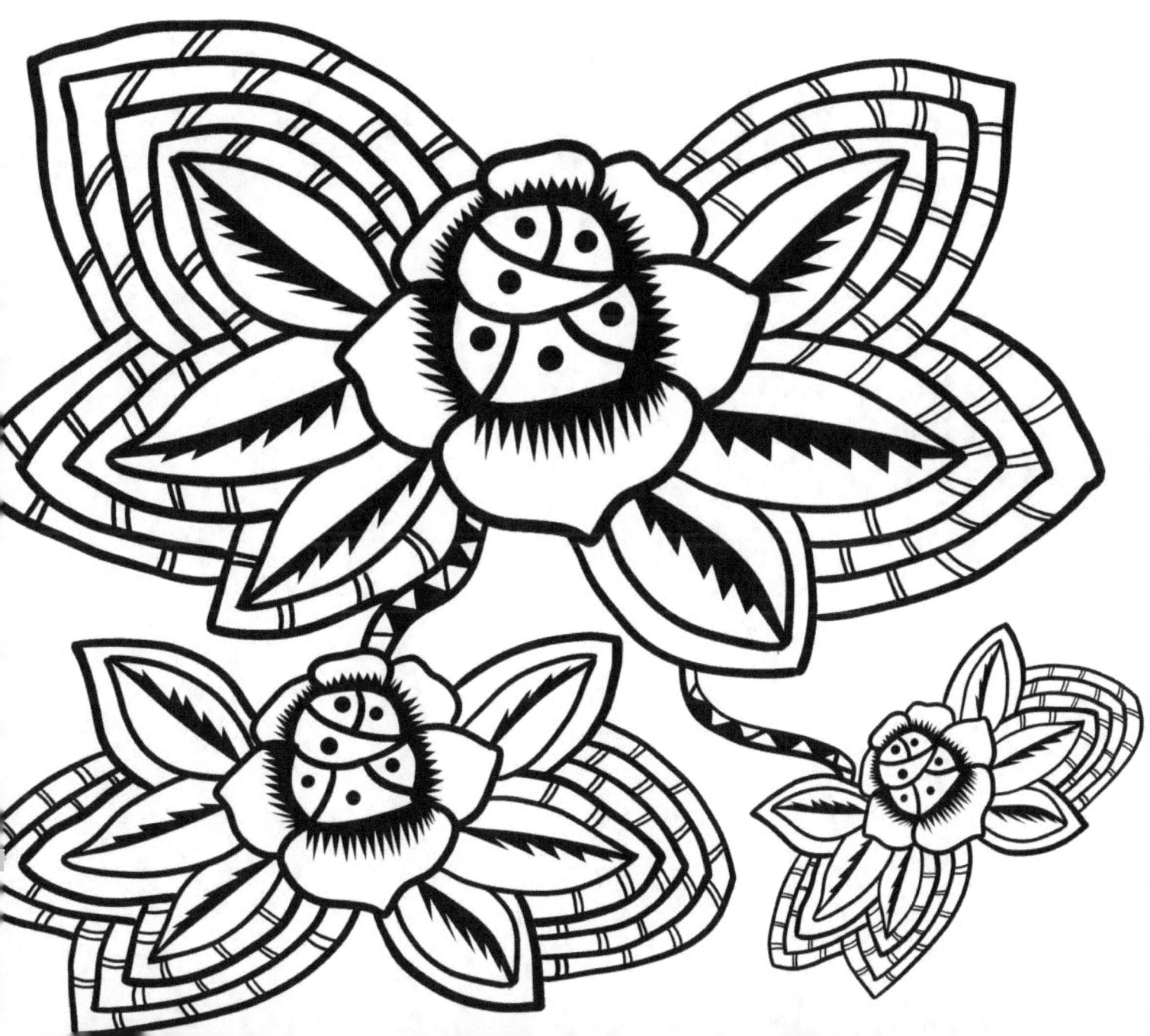

Yes, I'm A Nurse. No, I Don't Want To See It

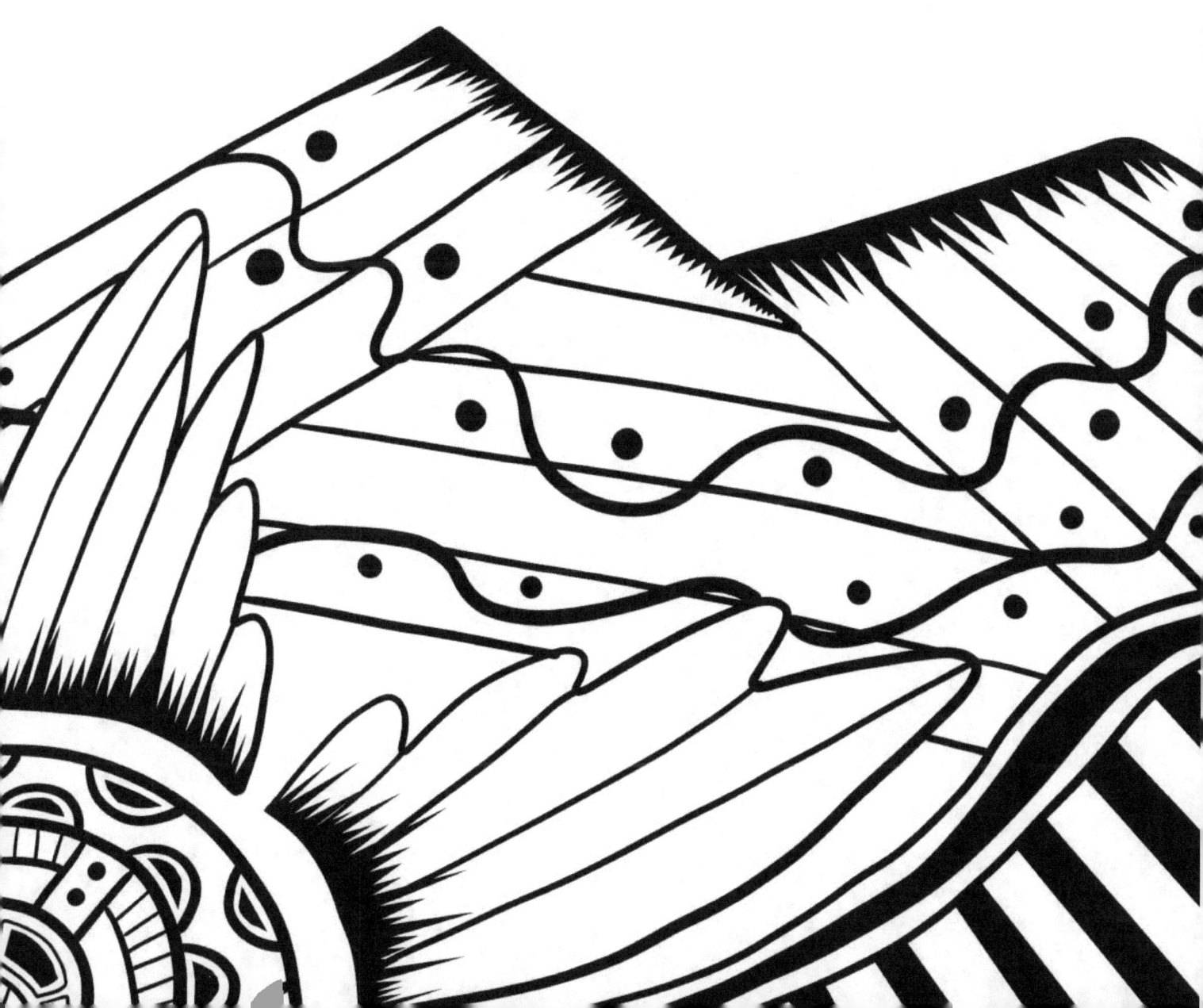